CHAIR YOGA FOR SENIOR OVER 60

A Complete 28 Days Challenge Guide To Weight Loss, Mobility, And Strength Exercises In Just 10 Minutes A Day To Transform And Improve Your Life

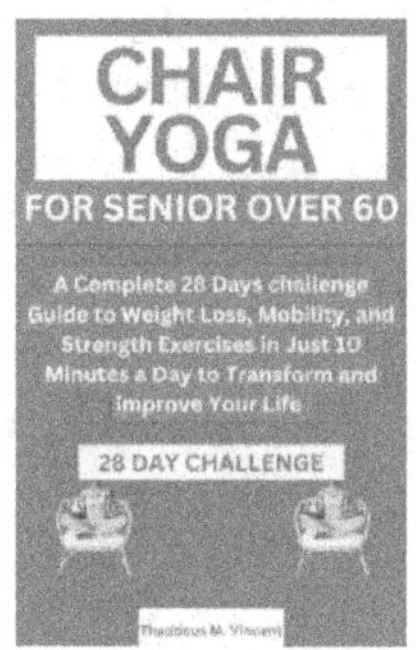

Thaddeus M. Vincent

Copyright © 2024 by Thaddeus M. Vincent

INTRODUCTION

As you settle into your preferred chair, feeling the weight of years in your bones, you consider the way it was once easy to transport, to stretch, to attain for the sky. But time has a way of catching up with us all, would not it?

Yet, there may be a glimmer of hope, a whisper of trade within the air. It comes within the form of a book, a manual to Chair Yoga for seniors such as you, over 60, seeking a manner to reclaim a piece of that flexibility, that power, that zest for lifestyles.

Opening the book, you're greeted by way of warm, inviting phrases, like an old pal welcoming you domestic. The pages are filled with gentle poses, each one tailored to suit your desires, your abilities. You study that Chair Yoga is not about contorting your body into not possible shapes; it is about finding movement, finding peace, finding yourself once more.

The advantages of Chair Yoga begin to unfold before your eyes. You examine approximately advanced flexibility, superior stability, and strengthened muscular tissues.

But it is not just your body that stands to benefit; your mind, too, can locate solace inside the rhythmic waft of breath and motion. Stress melts away, worries fade into the background, and you are left with a sense of calm, of centeredness, of being precisely wherein you want to be in this moment.

With every flip of the page, you find out new poses to strive, each one followed via clean instructions and useful illustrations. There's the gentle twist to ease anxiety for your backbone, the uplifting stretch to awaken your weary muscle tissues, and the soothing rest pose to lull you right into a nation of pleased tranquility.

And the first-rate part? You can do all of it from the comfort of your own chair, no fancy device or complex maneuvers required.

As you delve deeper into the ebook, you comprehend that Chair Yoga is greater than only a series of poses; it is a way of lifestyles. It teaches you to listen for your body, to honor its obstacles, and to have fun its victories, no matter how small they will seem.

It's approximately embracing the prevailing moment, locating pleasure in the easy act of breathing, of shifting, of being alive.

With each practice session, you sense yourself developing stronger, more resilient, more alive. You no longer dread the passage of time; rather, you welcome it with open fingers, understanding that with every passing day, you are becoming the quality version of yourself.

And as you close the book, a sense of gratitude washes over you, gratitude for the present of Chair Yoga, for the opportunity to reconnect along with your body, your mind, your spirit.

So as you sit there on your chair, basking in the glow of newfound power and energy, you can not assist but smile. For you've located the secret to growing older gracefully, to residing lifestyles to the fullest, to finding peace within the midst of chaos.

And all of it started out with a easy e-book, a manual to Chair Yoga for seniors like you, over 60, geared up to include the adventure with open palms and an open coronary heart.

CHAPTER 1:
UNDERSTANDING CHAIR YOGA

Origins And History Of Chair Yoga

Chair yoga originated from the principles of traditional hatha yoga and was specifically designed to deal with the physical limitations of practitioners.

Yoga teachers are concept to have first experimented with pose changes in the overdue twentieth century to facilitate college students who had been unable to execute them on a yoga mat.

As yoga's severa health advantages got here to be stated, the perception won traction, resulting within the introduction of specialized chair yoga packages and training. Presently, chair yoga is a dynamic discipline that is constantly evolving as instructors and practitioners adapt strategies and methods to house the necessities of diverse populations.

What Is Chair Yoga?

Chair yoga is an opportunity method to yoga wherein conventional yoga postures and exercises are modified to be executed with t

he help of a chair or even as seated in a single. It offers an method to yoga this is greater slight, rendering it available to folks who, via virtue of age, damage, or other constraints, might also have mobility problems or conflict with appearing conventional yoga poses.

Chair yoga includes the execution of changed iterations of poses through participants, with an emphasis on strengthening exercises, respiration techniques, and slight stretches. Due to its extreme adaptability, the exercise is appropriate for people of every age and ranges of health.

Benefits Of Chair Yoga For Seniors:

Seniors can gain from chair yoga in numerous approaches, which makes it a super form of relaxation and exercise for this population. In the first location, it enhances mobility and flexibility by gradually stretching the joints and muscle groups, thereby growing variety of motion and reducing stiffness.

In addition, chair yoga promotes electricity improvement, particularly within the palms, legs, and torso, that could help seniors in maintaining their independence and preventing falls.

In addition, the practice emphasizes relaxation strategies and deep breathing, all of which have the capability to relieve tension, decorate cognitive acuity, and promote holistic fitness. In addition, the exercise of chair yoga in a group environment fosters social bonds and a feel of community the various aged.

Common Concerns And Misconceptions

Concerns or misconceptions may be expressed regarding chair yoga, notwithstanding its manifold blessings, especially amongst aged people lacking familiarity with the technique.

The perception that chair yoga is much less powerful than conventional yoga or different styles of exercising is a typical fallacy.

Nevertheless, chair yoga gives similar advantages to conventional yoga, along with more suitable flexibility, energy, and relaxation, albeit with a reduced emphasis on intensity and extra accessibility. The possibility that chair yoga is insufficiently difficult or too easy for seniors conversant in more strenuous types of exercise is an extra issue.

Although chair yoga is characterised by using its mild nature, it stays amenable to customization according to character abilities and necessities, as there are picks to decorate the extent of intensity.

As a end result of its mild and approachable nature, chair yoga affords a multitude of bodily, mental, and emotional benefits for seniors over the age of sixty.

By comprehending its inception, blessings, and dispelling general fallacies, senior citizens can greater readily undertake chair yoga as a beneficial supplement to their well being regimen.

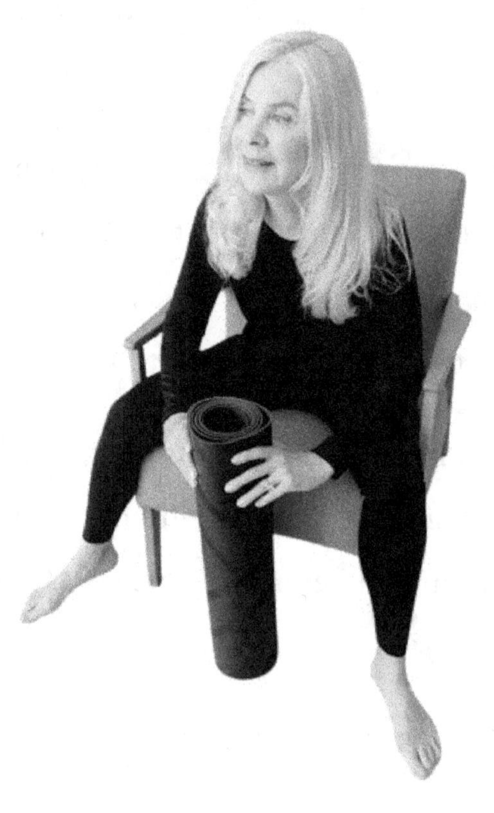

CHAPTER 2: INTRODUCTION TO CHAIR YOGA

Setting Up Your Space:

Prior to starting chair yoga for seniors over the age of 60, it's miles critical to put together the suitable area. Select a area that is sufficiently capacious to accommodate the chair without impeding its motion.

Remove out of your path any fixtures or items that might hinder your actions. Before starting the exercise, make certain that the chair is supported by using a stable surface to save you it from toppling over.

Creating an environment this is tranquil and serene can also serve to enhance the yoga revel in. Consider illuminating candles or playing gentle music to promote rest and concentration.

Selecting An Appropriate Chair:

An effective and stable chair yoga exercise requires careful consideration of the chair in query. For added assist, pick out a sturdy chair with a directly returned and armrests.

Wheeled or low-to-the-ground chairs need to be averted, as they will compromise balance. It have to no longer be hard to stay inside the chair for an prolonged time frame without experiencing pressure or pain.

Furthermore, guarantee that the chair facilitates suitable spinal and pelvic alignment at some point of the yoga postures. Add extra blankets or cushions if had to provide in addition help and comfort.

Equipment And Garments:

Incorporating appropriate apparel and making use of right apparatus can appreciably augment one's revel in of chair yoga. Select garments which might be breathable, loose-fitting, and permit unrestricted movement.

Garments which can be excessively snug or constricting must be prevented, as they can restrict one's range of movement. In addition, contemplate the usage of props—which includes yoga blocks, harnesses, or bolsters—to adapt poses and offer essential help.

Utilizing these helps during practice can aid in the enhancement of balance, stability, and alignment. Maintain hydration all through the consultation through maintaining a water bottle close by, specifically if training for an extended length.

Safety Precautions And Considerations:

It is especially essential that seniors over the age of 60 prioritize protection whilst performing chair yoga. Commence regularly even as final attuned on your body's cues, refraining from any motions that induce ache or misery.

As required, adjust poses to house the abilities and barriers of the character.During postures, maintain conscious control of your respiration and chorus from conserving it, as this can exacerbate anxiety and pressure. Before commencing chair yoga, individuals with pre-present scientific conditions or injuries ought to refer to a healthcare expert.

Furthermore, hold consciousness of any symptoms of imbalance, dizziness, or lightheadedness, and take essential pauses to rehydrate and relaxation. Lastly, technique chair yoga with self-compassion, patience, and kindness, always retaining in thoughts your body's particular necessities and limitations.

Seniors elderly 60 and above can properly and efficaciously experience the manifold advantages of chair yoga by using adhering to the subsequent tips: putting in their environment, deciding on the correct chair, obtaining suitable apparel and equipment, and placing safety precautions first.

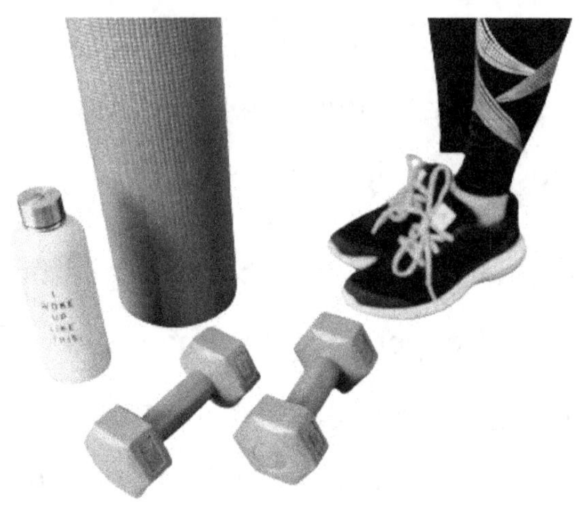

CHAPTER 3: FUNDAMENTAL CHAIR YOGA POSES

Warm-Up Positions:

In chair yoga for seniors over 60, it's far crucial first of all heat-up poses that prepare the frame and mind for the following exercise. Typically, those postures embody nuanced motions supposed to stimulate circulate, alleviate muscular anxiety, and rouse the joints.

An illustration of a warm-up pose is the seated neck roll, in which the practitioner tenderly and circumferentially rolls the neck, thereby alleviating tension and enhancing flexibility in the shoulders and neck.

Shoulder rolls are a further heat-up pose wherein elders roll their shoulders backwards and forwards, thereby increasing upper frame mobility and assuaging anxiety. By incorporating those heat-up poses into their chair yoga recurring, seniors can lessen their chance of damage at the same time as concurrently improving stream and flexibility.

Extended Stretches While Seated

Seated stretches are fundamental chair yoga positions that focus on the enhancement of physical flexibility and range of movement, with a specific emphasis on senior citizens aged 60 and above who may additionally encounter rigidity or limited mobility.

By requiring individuals to remain seated in a chair, those stretches make sure that people with mobility impairments or equilibrium worries can appropriately and effortlessly have interaction in them. The seated ahead bend is a often done seated exercising wherein seniors bend forward gently from the hips, extending their attain toward their feet or shins. This stretch assists in elongating the backbone, relieving lower again tension, and stretching the hamstrings.

An extra seated stretch is the seated side bend, which is achieved through extending one arm aloft and leaning lightly to the side to stretch the facet of the frame. For the elderly, seated stretches in chair yoga enhance flexibility, promote relaxation, and improve average health.

Stability And Equilibrium Poses:

In addition to decreasing the risk of falls, balance and balance poses are essential additives of chair yoga for seniors over 60, as they give a boost to balance, coordination, and confidence.

These postures were adjusted to be carried out in a steady way whilst seated or using the chair for support. The seated tree posture is an example of a balance pose in which an elderly character locations one foot at the ground whilst raising the alternative foot to relaxation at the inner thigh or calf.

In addition to testing equilibrium and stability, this pose complements awareness and attention. Stained knee lifts are an extra stability pose in which seniors raise one knee towards their torso even as maintaining an erect spine and tasty the center muscular tissues.

Through the implementation of stability and balance poses in chair yoga, senior citizens have the opportunity to improve their universal balance, mitigate the likelihood of falls, and preserve autonomy of their routine obligations.

Relaxing Postures Encompass:

For senior residents over the age of 60 to practice chair yoga and obtain anxiety alleviation, relaxation, and a feel of well-being, rest poses are vital. The reason of those poses is to facilitate profound relaxation through the release of physical tension and the promotion of intellectual tranquility.

Seniors who have interaction in seated meditation accomplish that at the same time as seated conveniently in a chair with their eyes closed, directing their interest in the direction of their breathing and permitting their mind to pass without important assessment.

 This sincere workout induces a state of relaxation, diminishes feelings of anxiety, and complements cognitive acuity. An extra rest pose is the seated forward fold with guide, wherein seniors guide their head on a cushion or block while gently folding ahead over their thighs. In addition to relieving stress from the again, shoulders, and neck, this pose encourages a feel of launch and surrender. The integration of relaxation poses into the chair yoga routine can cause enhanced tranquility, relaxation, and holistic fitness among senior residents.

End, chair yoga gives seniors over the age of 60 with a easy and handy technique of enhancing their bodily and mental nicely-being. The flexibility, energy, stability, and typical well-being of seniors can be stepped forward thru the mixing of various yoga sequences, inclusive of warm-up poses, seated stretches, mild twists and spinal movements, stability and balance poses, and relaxation poses.

The senior populace can derive severa benefits from chair yoga, which include more desirable high-quality of life, decreased anxiety, and multiplied relaxation. Seniors can maintain a wholesome and lively life-style while having access to the numerous benefits of chair yoga through consistent exercise.

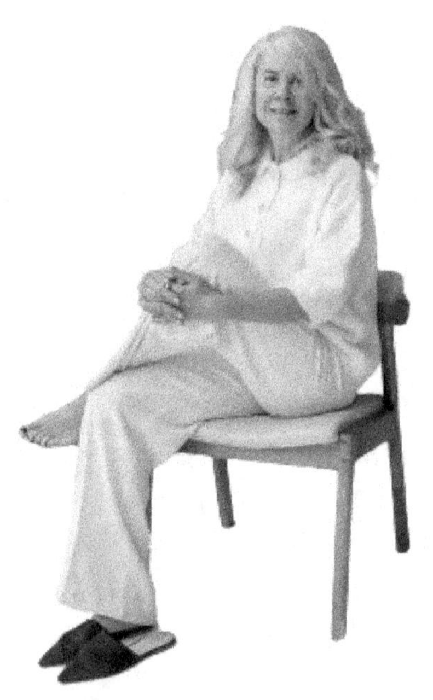

CHAPTER 4: TECHNIQUES OF BREATHING (PRANAYAMA)

Awareness Of One's Breath Is Important:

Particularly essential is breath consciousness for senior residents appearing chair yoga. It needs attention at the natural passage of the breath, specially on every exhalation and inhalation. Seniors can beautify the thoughts-body connection at some stage in yoga practice by using incorporating mindfulness into their moves via the incorporation of breath attention.

Seniors can also discover this heightened consciousness useful for tension reduction, relaxation, and the advertising of a tranquil disposition. Additionally, respiration cognizance promotes improved body oxygenation, which enhances vitality and basic fitness. This enables an more advantageous understanding of pranayama strategies, thereby empowering senior residents to optimize the benefits in their yoga routine.

Basic Breathing Methods:

Seat yoga for people elderly 60 and above is based on primary respiratory strategies. These physical games are clean to perform at the same time as located quite simply in a chair, are gentle, and are handy.

An instance of such an exercise is belly respiration, in which elderly people exhale progressively through the mouth while contracting the abdomen lightly and inhale deeply through the nostrils, allowing the abdomen to expand completely.

Seniors can further sell balance and relaxation through conducting same respiratory, which includes an same matter of inhalation and exhalation. By acting these trustworthy respiratory sporting activities, aged individuals can boom their lung potential, lower their anxiety, and improve their widespread sense of properly-being.

Pranayama's Advantages For Seniors:

The implementation of yogic respiratory techniques, or pranayama, into chair yoga regimens can offer seniors with a mess of blessings. Pranayama techniques resource inside the control of anxiety and anxiety among senior residents by way of stimulating the rest response of the body.

The parasympathetic apprehensive machine is inspired by deep breathing, which reduces the heartbeat fee and blood strain. In addition, pranayama improves oxygen flow all through the frame and strengthens the airlines, thereby enhancing respiratory characteristic. This is especially superb for aged folks that, as they age, may expand breathing headaches or diminished pulmonary feature.

Additional benefits of pranayama consist of greater cognitive feature, stepped forward sleep fine, and improved ordinary energy, all of which make a contribution to an better high-quality of existence for older adults.

Implementing Breath Work Into Everyday Life:

Seniors ought to include breath work into their everyday lives with a purpose to derive advantages that extend past the practice of yoga. The implementation of basic mindfulness practices, which includes conducting some deep breaths prior to meals or in reaction to emotions of hysteria, can assist aged individuals in developing a state of tranquility and attentiveness over the direction of the day.

Promoting the mixing of mindful respiration practices into habitual duties, inclusive of gardening or strolling, can moreover bolster the physical and intellectual energy of older adults. In addition, even a short each day practice of pranayama strategies for a couple of minutes can have vast wonderful influences at the bodily and mental properly-being of aged people.

By incorporating breath work into their every day routines, senior citizens can experience elevated ordinary resilience, decreased anxiety, and stronger strength ranges whilst faced with the challenges of lifestyles.

Breathe focus, basic respiratory sporting activities, pranayama strategies, and the incorporation of breath work into each day lifestyles are, in précis, critical elements of chair yoga designed for people aged 60 and above.

Seniors can reap better physical health, progressed mental properly-being, and a heightened experience of power with the implementation of those techniques. Seniors can live happier, healthier lives by means of harnessing the power in their respiratory through normal exercise and mindfulness.

CHAPTER 5: ROUTINES FOR CHAIR YOGA

A Brief Daily Schedule For Novices:

This chair yoga routine is specifically tailored for seniors elderly 60 and above who're inexperienced inside the exercise of yoga or have bodily limitations that restriction their mobility.

It emphasizes light motions to decorate energy, flexibility, and general health. Beginning the habitual are deep breathing sports that soothe the frame and promote mental clarity.

Subsequently, primary seated stretches concentrate on prominent muscle businesses, including the neck, shoulders, hands, and returned, thereby enhancing variety of motion and diminishing muscular tension.

Due to their accessibility and gentleness, these stretches are suitable for novices. Following this, the contributors engage in a quick rest exercise to re-set up their power degrees prior to continuing with their daily sports.

This senior-friendly daily routine serves as an exemplary initiation to chair yoga, offering a gradual and compotent practice of mindfulness and bodily pastime.

A Relaxing Morning Wake-Up Regimen:

This seated yoga routine is right for seniors over the age of 60 who wish to start the day with vigor and electricity. Gentle seated rotations and aspect stretches are carried out initially to stimulate the spine and decorate flow.

These sporting activities aid within the discount of muscle stress and anxiety that can have built up during the night time, whilst also priming the body for the following day. In order to growth alertness and oxygenate the frame, members perform energizing breathing sporting activities, consisting of deep inhales and exhales, after completing the stretches.

Additionally, the regimen consists of simple seated sun salutations, which foster flexibility and vitality. By integrating meditative movements and deep respiration into their morning recurring, senior citizens set up a optimistic surroundings that invigorates them and empowers them to confront the day's demanding situations.

Energizing Pick-Me-Up Routine Inside The Afternoon:

Especially amongst seniors elderly 60 and above, electricity tiers have a tendency to decrease during the route of the day. This chair yoga ordinary offers a revitalizing midday respite that complements both power degrees and awareness.

The recurring commences with revitalizing seated stretches and moderate twists, which serve to alleviate strain and decorate blood drift. These exercises aid inside the mitigation of fatigue and enhance cognitive acuity.

After completing the calisthenics, the individuals continue to carry out dynamic breathing physical activities, together with Kapalabhati (cranium shining breath), that are designed to invigorate the body and stimulate the worried system.

Flowing movements, which include arm circles and seated cat-cow stretches, also are integrated into the recurring for you to stimulate the senses and decorate posture. Seniors can breathe new existence into the the rest of the day by using devoting a few minutes to this invigorating routine.

This will allow them to confront the day with restored strength and vitality.

Wind-Down Relaxing Evening Routine:

It is crucial for seniors over the age of 60 to unwind and make arrangements for a restful night time's shut eye as the day draws to a near. This chair yoga routine promotes rest and anxiety comfort through the use of deep breathing and gentle actions.

It commences with mild shoulder rolls and seated ahead folds as a way of relieving daylong tension. These physical activities promote physical relaxation and facilitate the release of any residual tension.

Subsequent to the calisthenics, the contributors partake in tranquilizing breathing exercises, which include trade nose respiration, with the intention of alleviating anxiety and fostering a state of peace. Restorative postures, together with supported seated twists and legs up the chair, are incorporated into the recurring to promote profound rest and top the body for shut eye.

By integrating this calming night routine into their nocturnal routine, aged people can enhance the high-quality in their sleep and general nation of fitness.

This regimen gives a methodical framework for integrating chair yoga into one's every day habitual, encompassing an collection of techniques that accommodate various necessities and inclinations.

Seniors can benefit from chair yoga in quite a few approaches, inclusive of a slight morning wake-up habitual, an afternoon select-me-up, and an evening relaxation. Among the various advantages

of chair yoga are more suitable flexibility, energy,
and mental health.

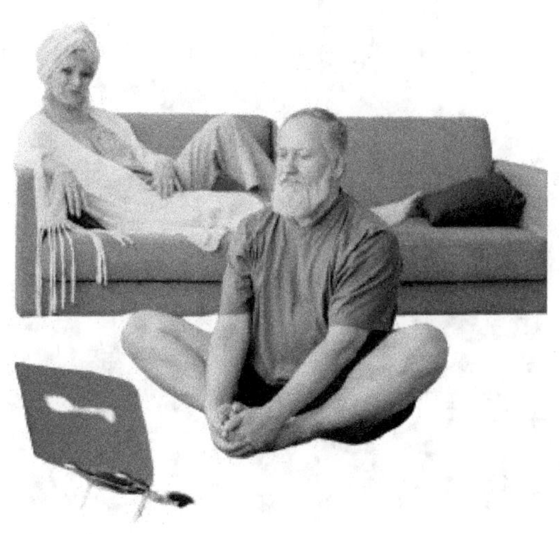

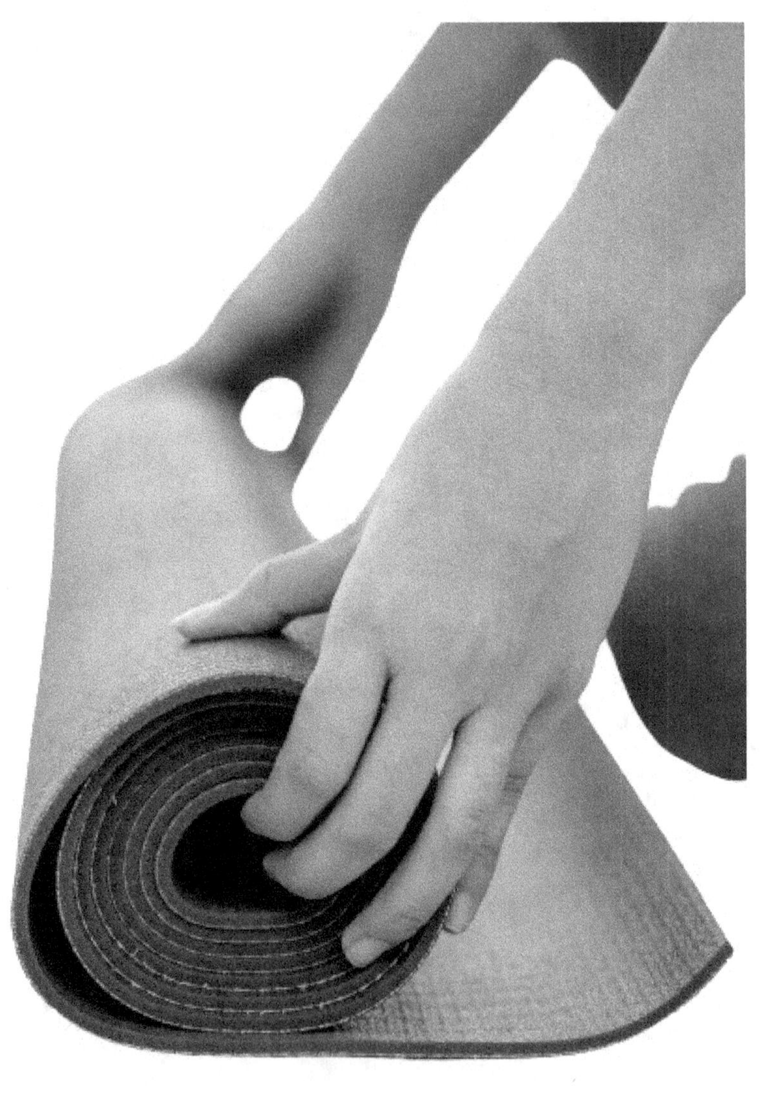

CHAPTER 6:
INCORPORATING CHAIR YOGA INTO YOUR LIFESTYLE

Chair Yoga For Optimal Lifestyle:

Chair yoga is an adapted variant of the conventional yoga poses that calls for the practitioner to maintain a seated position or utilize a chair for help.

Seniors over the age of 60 who may additionally have mobility problems or different bodily boundaries can advantage from its numerous benefits. By supplying a low-effect method of physical pastime, chair yoga can help seniors in keeping an energetic physique.

By incorporating respiration sporting activities, meditation strategies, and slight stretches, chair yoga complements muscularity, equilibrium, and flexibility. Through the mixing of chair yoga into their daily routine, senior citizens may also potentially study upgrades in their strength degrees, joint stress, and move.

This physically on hand forms of exercising permits older people, regardless of their bodily circumstance or limitations, to stay lively and experience the advantages of yoga.

Chair Yoga For Anxiety And Stress Management:

Managing anxiety and anxiety is critical for the overall health of seniors, who're especially vulnerable to the problems that accompany getting old. Chair yoga offers convenient integration of pressure-relieving and relaxation techniques that are fairly powerful. By engaging in mindful meditation, deep breathing exercises, and mild stretches, chair yoga assists seniors in assuaging strain, selling intellectual tranquility, and cultivating an internal experience of concord.

Regular chair yoga practice can assist seniors in growing more effective stress control talents, assuaging anxiety, and improving their usual mental nicely-being. In search of tranquility and equilibrium, chair yoga is an excellent practice for seniors due to its approachable nature.

Practicing Chair Yoga To Enhance Posture And Mobility:

Seniors must maintain exquisite mobility and posture on the way to remain active and independent as they age. Chair yoga includes a chain of low-depth stretches and sports which might be intended to beautify mobility, flexibility, and posture.

Seniors can reduce their danger of falls and accidents by strengthening the muscle mass that guide correct posture and alignment through steady chair yoga exercise.

Additionally, chair yoga improves joint mobility and range of movement, allowing seniors to perform every day duties with self belief and luxury. On and off the chair, chair yoga encourages seniors to keep a sturdy, solid, and balanced posture through the cultivation of frame attention and right alignment.

Consequently, elderly people can revel in more suitable physical function, decreased pain and misery, and stepped forward mobility, all of which empower them to completely have interaction in life.

Chair Yoga For Improved Rest:

Numerous seniors aged 60 and above experience sleep disturbances, along with insomnia and difficulty last unconscious all night. Chair yoga affords a variety of effective but sensitive strategies that encourage restful sleep and enhance the overall great of sleep.

Seniors can set up a relaxing twilight ordinary that communicates to their body and thoughts the need for relaxation via conducting respiration exercises and rest poses previous to sleep. By facilitating rest, assuaging physical tension, and calming the mind, chair yoga assists seniors in falling asleep and ultimate subconscious for the duration of the night.

By integrating chair yoga into their evening regimen, senior residents may be capable of gain a more profound and uninterrupted shut eye, thereby augmenting their power and improving their fashionable nation of health and well-being.

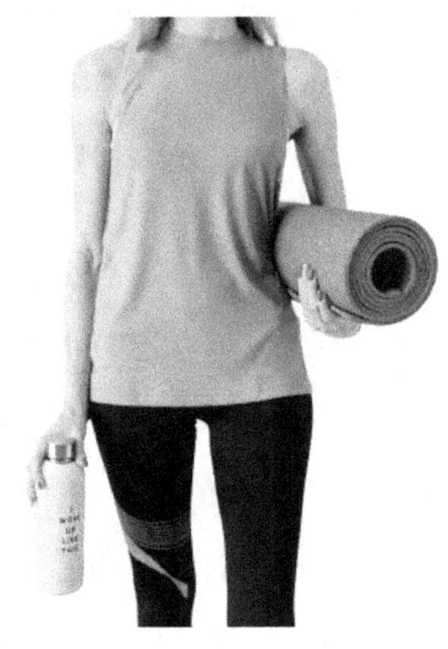

CHAPTER 7: MEDITATION AND MINDFULNESS CONTAIN

An Overview Of Mindfulness:

Mindfulness is the field of directing one's entire attention to the existing second without passing judgment. It includes maintaining whole awareness of both internal and outside instances, without preoccupation with regrettable recollections or anxieties regarding the destiny.

Mindfulness may be mainly nice for seniors over the age of 60, because it promotes the improvement of a tranquil country of thoughts, mitigates anxiety, and complements usual health. A multitude of strategies may be employed to cultivate mindfulness, encompassing mindful motion, frame exams, conscious breathing, and chair yoga.

Straightforward Meditation Methods:

Seniors can correctly domesticate mindfulness and improve their intellectual and physical health through the exercise of meditation. Older adults can engage in a variety of honest meditation techniques from the ease of a chair.

A approach that includes directing one's attention toward the feeling of breath entering and exiting the frame is referred to as "focused respiratory." An extra technique is guided imagery, wherein elderly people visualize themselves in a placid and tranquil putting, thereby facilitating rest and unwinding.

Body experiment meditation promotes rest and body focus via the systematic attention on various body regions. By accommodating the needs and capabilities of senior residents, those strategies emerge as on hand and high quality for all individuals.

Advantages Of Meditation For The Elderly:

Numerous and good sized are the benefits of meditation for seniors. To begin with, meditation aids inside the relief of tension and tension, each of which can be regularly occurring difficulties encountered by a great range of aged individuals.

Regular mindfulness meditation exercise can teach seniors to more successfully control tension and induce a heightened feel of serenity and peace. In addition, reminiscence and cognitive function, each of which might be vital for best ageing, may be improved thru meditation.

Additionally, seniors who meditate may additionally revel in advanced temper, sleep, and normal health. Moreover, studies has confirmed that meditation confers physical advantages, together with reduced arterial strain, alleviated inflammation, and better immune device function. Incorporating meditation into their daily exercises can extensively enhance the exceptional of existence for individuals who are 60 years of age or older.

Implementing Mindfulness Into Everyday Life:

In addition to carrying out dependent meditation routines, aged individuals have the capability to foster mindfulness at some point of their ordinary lives with the aid of using truthful yet impactful strategies.

Adopting conscious ingesting, wherein seniors consciousness intently on the taste, texture, and sensations of every morsel of meals, can facilitate this aim. By cultivating a heightened experience of gratitude for nourishment, seniors also can encourage the adoption of more healthy dietary practices.

Seniors can similarly develop their mindfulness through conducting mindful strolling, for the duration of which they concentrate on the sensations of every step, the encompassing attractions and sounds, and the rhythm of their respiratory.

Participating in endeavors along with painting, gardening, or taking note of music can serve as additional occasions to domesticate mindfulness and presence.

The incorporation of mindfulness practices into the everyday lives of seniors can result in better ranges of satisfaction, fortitude, and happiness.

In summary, mindfulness and meditation provide extensive benefits for people aged 60 and above, enhancing their bodily fitness, mental state, and average popular of residing.

Seniors can live with a renewed sense of energy and motive, find out more peace and contentment, and improve their ability to deal with the demanding situations of growing older by means of integrating simple meditation techniques and cultivating mindfulness into their daily lives.

CHAPTER 8: 28 DAY CHAIR YOGA CHALLENGE

Here's a 28-day Chair Yoga Challenge that goals to infuse your days with tranquility, power, and a renewed experience of connection in your body and thoughts. Each day builds upon the last, guiding you thru a adventure of self-discovery and mild movement. Let's begin:

Day 1: Grounding Breath:

Start by using sitting quite simply for your chair, feet flat at the ground. Close your eyes and take 5 deep breaths, feeling the feeling of the breath filling your lungs. With every exhale, believe releasing any anxiety or pressure from your body.

Practice: five minutes

Day 2: Neck Release:

Gently tilt your head to the right, bringing your ear in the direction of your shoulder. Hold for some breaths, and then transfer to the left aspect. Repeat three times on each side, specializing in releasing anxiety in the neck and shoulders.

Practice: three minutes

Day 3: Seated Cat-Cow:

Place your hands on your knees. As you inhale, arch your lower back and raise your chest (Cow Pose). As you exhale, round your spine and tuck your chin in the direction of your chest (Cat Pose). Flow between these poses for five breaths, synchronizing movement with breath.

Practice: five minutes

Day 4 Shoulder Rolls:

Sit tall together with your arms by means of your facets. Inhale as you elevate your shoulders toward your ears, then exhale and roll them back and down. Repeat for 10 rounds, feeling every roll release tension inside the shoulders.

Practice: three mins

Day 5: Spinal Twist

Cross your proper hand for your left knee and location your left hand at the lower back of the chair. Inhale to prolong your spine, then exhale to curl lightly to the left. Hold for 3 breaths, then switch aspects. Repeat two times on each aspect.

Practice: 5 mins

Day 6: Seated Forward Fold Sit toward the the front of your chair with feet hip-width aside. Hinge at your hips and fold ahead, letting your arms dangle in the direction of the ground. Relax your neck and breathe deeply for 5 breaths, feeling the stretch to your hamstrings and decrease returned.

Practice: five mins

Day 7: Mindful Meditation

Take 10 minutes to take a seat quietly for your chair, focusing on your breath. Notice the feeling of each inhale and exhale, permitting thoughts to come and move without judgment. Embrace the prevailing moment with gratitude and popularity.

Practice: 10 minutes

Day 8: Chest Opener

Interlace your fingers in the back of your back and lightly straighten your fingers as you elevate your chest closer to the ceiling. Take three deep breaths, feeling the stretch throughout the chest and shoulders.

Practice: 3 minutes

Day 9: Seated Sun Salutation

Flow via a changed Sun Salutation, reaching your hands overhead as you inhale, then folding forward as you exhale. Move slowly and with aim, connecting breath to movement for five rounds.

Practice: 7 mins

Day 10: Ankle Circles

Extend your proper leg and circle your ankle clockwise, then counterclockwise. Repeat at the left side. This simple movement helps enhance flow and mobility inside the ankles.

Practice: 3 mins

Day 11: Seated Mountain Pose

Sit tall with ft flat at the ground. Reach your palms overhead and press your hands together. Take 3 deep breaths, feeling grounded and energized like a mountain.

Practice: 3 minutes

Day 12: Hip Opener

Cross your right ankle over your left knee, flexing your proper foot. Gently press down on your proper knee to deepen the stretch to your right hip. Hold for 5 breaths, then transfer sides.

Practice: 5 minutes

Day 13: Chair Yoga Flow

Combine gentle moves like neck stretches, shoulder rolls, ahead folds, and twists into a flowing series. Move mindfully, following your breath and being attentive to your body's cues.

Practice: 10 minutes

Day 14: Gratitude Practice

Take a moment to reflect on three things you're grateful for today. Cultivating gratitude can shift your perspective and produce extra joy into your lifestyles.

Practice: 5 minutes

Day 15: Seated Side Stretch

Reach your right arm overhead and lean to the left, growing area alongside the right aspect of your frame. Hold for three breaths, then transfer sides. Feel the stretch alongside the facet frame and ribcage.

Practice: five mins

Day 16: Chair Yoga Nidra

Find a cushty seated position and close your eyes. Follow a guided Yoga Nidra meditation, allowing your frame and mind to go into a kingdom of deep relaxation and rejuvenation.

Practice: 15 minutes

Day 17: Mindful Eating Practice

aware ingesting at some stage in one meal these days. Slow down, appreciate every chew, and pay attention to the tastes, textures, and sensations in your frame.

Practice: 1 min

Day 18: Seated Heart Opener

Interlace your hands in the back of your again and raise your chest closer to the sky, establishing your heart area. Take 3 deep breaths, feeling a feel of vulnerability and braveness.

Practice: three minutes

Day 19: Chair Pigeon Pose

Cross your proper ankle over your left knee and flex your right foot. Lean forward barely, feeling a stretch on your right hip and outer thigh. Hold for five breaths, then switch aspects.

Practice: 5 minutes

Day 20: Breath Awareness

Take five minutes to study your breath with out looking to change it. Notice the rhythm, intensity, and fine of your breath because it moves inside and out of your body.

Practice: 5 minutes

Day 21: Seated Twist Variation

Sit tall and area your right hand at the back of the chair. Inhale to prolong your backbone, then exhale to curl gently to the right, setting your left hand on your proper knee. Hold for three breaths, then transfer sides.

Practice: five minutes

Day 22: Chair Yoga for Stress Relief

Practice a sequence of calming poses and deep breathing physical activities to lessen stress and sell relaxation. Allow yourself to permit go of tension and find peace within.

Practice: 10 minutes

Day 23: Seated Side Bend

Reach your proper arm overhead and lean to the left, developing a gentle stretch alongside the proper facet of your frame. Hold for five breaths, then transfer aspects. Feel the expansiveness and freedom for your torso.

Practice: five mins

Day 24: Chair Yoga for Better Posture

Focus on sitting tall with a lengthened spine at some point of the day. Practice gentle stretches and sports to strengthen your core muscle groups and help proper alignment.

Practice: 7 minutes

Day 25: Self-Compassion Practice

Offer yourself words of kindness and understanding, acknowledging that you are doing the best you could in this second. Treat yourself with the equal compassion you will provide to a dear buddy.

Practice: five minutes

Day 26: Seated Warrior Pose

Extend your proper leg out to the side and bend your left knee, planting your foot on the floor. Reach your fingers overhead and lean gently to the right, feeling a stretch alongside the left side of your body. Hold for three breaths, then transfer sides.

Practice: 5 minutes

Day 27: Chair Yoga for Better Sleep

Practice a calming bedtime ordinary that consists of gentle stretches, relaxation techniques, and deep respiratory sports to put together your frame and mind for a restful night's sleep.

Practice: 10 minutes

Day 28: Celebration And Reflection

Take a moment to rejoice your dedication to your chair yoga practice during the last 28 days. Reflect on any adjustments you've got observed in your body, thoughts, and spirit, and set intentions for persevering with your journey of self-care and self-discovery.

Congratulations on completing the 28-Day Chair Yoga Challenge! May the advantages of your exercise maintain to enhance your life in limitless ways.

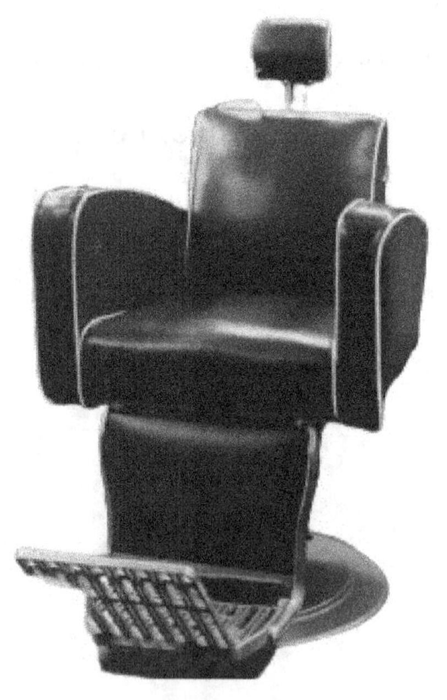

CHAPTER 9: ADVANCED CHAIR YOGA POSES (OPTIONAL)

Consolidating Your Practice:

To deepen one's exercise of chair yoga for seniors over 60, one need to development beyond the fundamental poses as a way to growth their flexibility, energy, and cognizance.

This may be accomplished via a number of strategies, consisting of the incorporation of meditation, the exercise of breathwork, and the exploration of more advanced asanas or poses.

By establishing a greater profound connection with your body, thoughts, and spirit, intensifying your exercise promotes internal serenity and properly-being. You can revel in extra physical and mental blessings, inclusive of greater balance, reduced tension, and multiplied vitality, via steadily advancing your practice.

Balance-Difficultating Poses:

Seniors must perform stability poses which will growth their balance and reduce their risk of falling. Compelling balance poses in chair yoga for seniors over the age of 60 may be adjusted to match the abilities of the individuals while retaining the pose's beneficial nature.

These postures may consist of seated balances that target alignment and engage the middle muscle groups, as well as status balances supported with the aid of the chair, such as warrior III or tree pose.

Regularly acting difficult balance poses can assist seniors improve their proprioception, coordination, and self-assurance of their bodily abilities, in the long run ensuing in multiplied independence and an greater pleasant of lifestyles.

Exercises For Building Strength:

Seniors have to engage in electricity-constructing sports to keep bone density, muscle tissues, and general purposeful independence. Incorporating strength-constructing physical games into chair yoga for seniors over 60 can function a counterbalance to the inherent decline in muscle energy and endurance that takes place with advancing age.

Utilizing body resistance or supplementary gadget along with resistance bands or mild weights, these sporting activities can target foremost muscle businesses including the legs, palms, middle, and again. Instances of sporting activities that decorate strength and power include spinal twists, chair squats, seated leg raises, and bicep curls.

Consistent implementation of those sports now not best enhances muscular strength however also promotes right alignment, posture, and overall mobility, thereby empowering aged individuals to maintain an active and took part-in lifestyle.

Alterations To Various Capabilities:

To make certain that chair yoga for seniors over 60 is accessible and inclusive for all individuals, it is vital to incorporate changes for various abilities. Potential adjustments that can be essential to accommodate mobility regulations, joint soreness, or continual ailments like arthritis or osteoporosis include enhancing poses.

For example, senior citizens who have limited mobility can also execute standing poses while seated or make use of extra support including blocks or bolsters. Moreover, instructors have the capability to offer alternative variations of poses a good way to accommodate the specific necessities of each student, permitting those with bodily barriers to partake within the therapeutic blessings of yoga.

Chair yoga training establish a nurturing atmosphere wherein seniors can securely have interaction inside the practice while additionally encountering the profound physiological and psychological benefits of yoga, by means of accommodating variations in performance ability.

In end, senior residents over the age of 60 who want to deepen their chair yoga practice must look at more advanced strategies that improve their flexibility, balance, power, and mindfulness. Strength-constructing physical games sell muscular patience and functional autonomy, whereas tough balance poses enhance posture and self-assurance. Adjustments to deal with people with varying competencies guarantee that every participant can interact in the hobby in a secure and green manner, promoting an environment of inclusiveness and empowerment.

By integrating these additives into their habitual, senior citizens can completely enjoy the advantages that chair yoga offers, together with enhanced bodily health, better intellectual acuity, and advanced emotional kingdom.

CHAPTER 10: FAQS AND TROUBLESHOOTING

Frequent Concerns Regarding Chair Yoga

Before determining to participate, many seniors, particularly the ones over the age of 60, may have inquiries about chair yoga. "What is chair yoga?" is a often asked inquiry. Chair yoga, that is practiced whilst seated on or using a chair for guide, is a modified shape of yoga.

The regimen integrates conscious respiration sporting events, stretching routines, and stretches. This particular style of yoga is well-appropriate for aged folks who can also revel in demanding situations with mobility or ascending and descending from the ground.

An additional often asked inquiry pertains to the suitability of chair yoga for senior residents who've health conditions. Adaptations can be made to deal with a number health conditions, consisting of but now not confined to arthritis, osteoporosis, and coronary heart disease.

Prior to starting a brand new workout regimen, seniors must, however, consult their healthcare provider to make sure that it's far secure and appropriate for his or her particular necessities.

Confronting Difficulties And Obstacles

There are strategies to be had to correctly triumph over the demanding situations or boundaries that seniors may face while beginning chair yoga.

Feeling self-conscious or humiliated whilst practicing yoga in a set is a common impediment. Seniors can surmount this undertaking through seeking out chair yoga lessons which can be tailor-made to their age or ability level, thereby fostering an environment conducive to consolation and help. An additional impediment is experiencing bodily soreness or anguish even as appearing unique poses.

Seniors have to pay close interest to their bodies and adjust their poses consequently in an effort to prevent stress or damage. Moreover, they may discover it difficult to maintain consistency and motivation in relation to chair yoga.

To surmount this assignment and set up chair yoga as a dependancy that endures, it is advisable to set up sensible objectives, domesticate a nurturing environment within one's family, and derive delight from the interest.

Guidance On Overcoming Unease Or Resistance

There exist multiple techniques that can be hired to beautify the accessibility and enjoyment of chair yoga for seniors who stumble upon resistance or distress during the practice.

One piece of advice is to increase the duration and depth of the practice incrementally as you progress. Seniors might also commence with lesser sessions and regularly expand them as their consolation and self assurance stage will increase. Seniors can also reduce tension and promote relaxation by way of concentrating at the breath and mindfulness components of chair yoga.

Additionally, the combination of relaxing and stretching techniques can aid in the mitigation of bodily tension and pain. Furthermore, so that you can acquire steering and encouragement, seniors may attain out to circle of relatives participants, associates, or a certified yoga instructor. In end, senior citizens have to exercise self-compassion and perseverance as they confront the barriers associated with starting a new exercising routine.

Seniors can develop a favorable rapport with chair yoga and progressively recognise its manifold benefits with the aid of embracing a compassionate and unbiased mindset towards themselves.

Summary

Concluding Remarks Of Encouragement:

When thinking about chair yoga for seniors over the age of 60, it's miles essential to well known the profound impact that consistency and commitment can have on a system of transformation. By engaging in regular practice, people have the ability to have a look at substantial upgrades of their physical health, intellectual kingdom, and typical excellent of existence.

Particularly encouraging is the truth that chair yoga may be modified to in shape the necessities and abilities of each character. There is always area for strengthen and development, no matter one's stage of experience, be it newbie or years. You will discover uncharted depths of staying power, flexibility, and power through drawing close every consultation with an open mind and a willingness to analyze your frame's potential.

Keep in mind that even the smallest progress represents a triumph deserving of jubilation, and that setbacks are merely activities for development and getting to know. It is critical to approach the adventure with a sense of curiosity, compassion, and persistence, as every on the spot spent at the mat represents an funding in a single's long-time period fitness.

Dedicating Yourself To Chair Yoga:

A dedication to chair yoga for seniors over the age of 60 requires a mental and prioritization adjustment, in place of in reality attending magnificence or practicing at home.

Primarily, it is critical to allocate specific time to your exercise, treating it with the identical diploma of importance as another issue of your each day routine. Determine a constant time that works for you, whether or not or not it's earlier than rest, during your lunch break, or first component within the morning.

Moreover, setting up an surroundings that is conducive to exercise can notably augment one's revel in. Establish a conducive surroundings without extraneous factors, making sure the presence of crucial furniture along with a strong chair, bolstering gadgets, and enough illumination. By enhancing your practice in response in your frame's signals, you may prioritize self-care.

 Should you be experiencing fatigue or discomfort, feel free to adjust poses or take pauses as vital. Keep in thoughts that progress is sluggish, and that consistent, deliberate attempt over the years often yields the hugest gains.

By dedicating oneself completely to the practice of chair yoga, one will gather an incalculable array of advantages, along with more desirable physical energy, advanced intellectual acuity, and reinforced emotional fortitude.

Conclusion

In conclusion, chair yoga isn't always pretty much physical movement; it's a journey in the direction of rejuvenation, vitality, and pleasure for seniors elderly 60 and above. It's approximately embracing the know-how of the years at the same time as nurturing your body, thoughts, and spirit in a gentle but profound way.

Through the easy act of sitting in a chair and transferring with intention, seniors can free up a world of benefits that amplify a ways beyond the bodily realm. Chair yoga gives a sanctuary in which you may reconnect with yourself , locating peace amidst life's hustle and bustle.

With every breath and stretch, you are not just firming muscle mass or improving flexibility; you're reclaiming your strength, reclaiming your joy, and reclaiming your existence. It's a practice that meets you wherein you're, honoring your unique adventure and guiding you closer to a brighter, extra vibrant destiny.

So, permit go of any doubts or reservations, and embody the beauty of chair yoga. Let it be your partner at the route to wellness, helping you navigate the challenges of growing older with grace and resilience.

Remember, it's never too overdue to begin, and each motion brings you in the direction of a existence packed with vitality, balance, and serenity. Let chair yoga be your gateway to an extra colorful, empowered, and pleasurable life.

www.ingramcontent.com/pod-product-compliance
Lightning Source LLC
Chambersburg PA
CBHW061256250726
48653CB00002B/671